Finally, Free!

Gwendolyn Littleton White

DEDICATION

This book is dedicated to Mikasha White Hawk, Shellie White Draper, Madison Amaryl Hawk, Megan Alexandra Simmons, Casey Addison Draper, Cameron Miles Draper, Charles Nathaniel Hawk, II, and Anthony Pichone Draper for being a loving supportive family.

CONTENTS

INTRODUCTION

Gastro esophageal reflux is a disease that affects more than 50 million Americans.

The prevalence of acid reflux experienced at least once a week has increased by almost 50% over the past decade, NTNU (Norwegian University of Science and Technology) researchers report in a long term study of almost 80,000 people published online in Gut. Women seem to be more vulnerable to developing the condition than men. The rise in prevalence of acid reflux may be partly explained by increasing rates of overweight and obesity, which are known risk factors for the condition, while the patterns seen in women might be down to the use of hormone replacement therapy. But they warn: "The increasing prevalence of [acid reflux] is alarming, because it will most likely contribute to the increasing incidence of adenocarcinoma of the esophagus in the western population."(Ness-Jensen, Lindam, Lagergren, & Hveem, 2012)

This book gives my account, as one of the 50 million Americans who have been affected by GERD, of the acid reflux disease. I will give details of the prevalence of acid reflux in my life for more than twenty years, which has led to the more serious form, GERD. I tell how I used a dramatic new approach proposed by a microbiologist (Norm Robillard, Ph.D.), to stop my acid reflux; after having suffered extensively from GERD for most of my adult life. And, like Dr. Robillard, I can speak from first hand knowledge about the effectiveness of this new approach, which is completely different from the medical treatment that I have received for more than twenty years.

In writing this book, I have three goals: 1. To encourage those who suffer with reflux to get some treatment. Don't allow the condition go untreated for any length of time because this gives way to more severe issue. The consequences could be GERD or even more complicated, Barrett's. 2. To describe how I used the step-by-step process to eliminate my acid reflux. 3. Show GERD sufferers how to implement the four-step process to make the life altering change from a high carbohydrate diet to a very low carb diet with ease; which will set them free from acid reflux. This book will can be their ace in the hole.

1 MY EXPERIENCE WITH ACID REFLUX

In this first chapter, I give an overview of my experience as one of the 50 million Americans who have been affected by GERD. I will give details of the prevalence of acid reflux in my life for more than twenty years, which has led to the more serious form, GERD.

I have had GERD for more than twenty years. And before that, I suffered from untreated acid reflux. This disease has affected both my health and quality of life. Initially, I didn't seek treatment because I didn't know about acid reflux. I had not ever heard of it. Indigestion, on the other hand, was something that I understood and recognized its symptoms. I knew that it was a common occurrence for many Americans. But, I didn't realize that it could also be a sign of an underlying medical issue that should be taken seriously.

During the early stages, I tried to clean up my diet to avoid the trigger foods that caused indigestion by limiting processed foods and increasing my intake of fruits and vegetables to help reduce chances of indigestion. Perhaps, this attributed to the periods when I had no recurrence of acid reflux.

My symptoms (acid reflux) gradually worsened and this took me in for treatment, on occasion, to the emergency room. In each instance, the physician recommended proton pump inhibitors (acid reducing drugs) as treatment. "Essentially, these drugs slam the brakes on the acid-producing pumps in your stomach, when you stop taking them that built-up acid can be unleashed with a vengeance." Unfortunately, these drugs failed to address the underlying causes of my acid reflux, while giving temporary relief. Instead, they compounded the issues and made them worse. I was never bothered with Globus hysrericus (a feeling of having a lump in the throat), but developed such symptoms after cessation of the PPIs. According to a new study, "Treatment with the anti-heartburn drugs known as proton pump inhibitors (PPIs) for eight weeks induces acid-related symptoms like heartburn, acid regurgitation and dyspepsia once treatment is withdrawn in healthy individuals." ("Why Stomach Acid Is Good For You DR. WRIGHT'S PRODUCTS," n.d.) ("Why You Should Get Off Prescription Acid-Reducing Drugs ASAP!" n.d.)

My condition went untreated for years and this eventually

led to the 2001 diagnosis, Barrett's. "Barrett's esophagus is a serious complication of GERD, which stands for gastro esophageal reflux disease. In Barrett's esophagus, normal tissue lining the esophagus -- the tube that carries food from the mouth to the stomach -- changes to tissue that resembles the lining of the intestine." Barrett's is a more serious condition in which the lower wall of the esophagus has been damaged by acid that overflows into the esophagus. I was first diagnosed with Barrett's in 2001 and this led me down a road of discovery and research that has culminated with this book. After the diagnosis, I was placed on daily doses of Protonix and Ranitidine. Two years later, I went back for a repeat endoscopy. The doctor was confounded. "Did I say you had Barrett's?" he asked. If only I had asked more questions. I assumed my condition was "no more Barrett's esophagus." based on the doctor's comment. Until this day, I don't know what he meant. Nevertheless, I continued my literacy campaign. I wanted to better understand the medicine and it's side affects in order that I could make informed choices. I studied and researched any and all literature that I could get my hands on about acid reflux and PPIs. According to recent studies, PPIs cause the very type of symptoms they are intended to prevent if you stop taking them. Dr. Jonathan Wright explains, "…Heartburn and GERD are almost always caused by a LACK of stomach acid, rather than an overproduction thereof. There are actually over 16,000 articles supporting the fact that suppressing stomach acid does not treat the problem. It only treats the symptoms. And one of the explanations for this is that when you suppress the amount of acid in your stomach, you decrease your body's ability to kill the bacteria. So it actually makes your condition worse and perpetuates the

problem." ("Why Stomach Acid Is Good For You DR.
WRIGHT'S PRODUCTS," n.d.).

Meanwhile, my symptoms had been held at bay for years.
But in 2012 the symptoms recurred. And they recurred with
a vengeance. This time I was afflicted with the worst bout of
reflux and GERD that I had ever known. Acid came through
my nostrils as I slept and I couldn't lie down without reflux.
I had pains in my chest, back and abdomen. My primary
care doctor prescribed pantoprazole and referred me to a
gastroenterologist. Meanwhile, I took the "big boys." This is
what she called the pantoprazole. I took them until I was
able to get in to see the gastroenterologist and have an
endoscopy.

2 THE TEST AND DIAGNOSIS

During the endoscopy, a capsule, approximately the size of a gel cap was temporarily attached to the wall of my esophagus. The purpose of the capsule was to measure pH levels in my esophagus and transmit this information wirelessly to a portable receiver I wore on my waistband for 48 hours. This was called a BRAVO, a pH test to help my doctor determine if I had acid reflux. This pH test was supposed to measure the degree of acidity or alkalinity in my esophagus. The test period lasted 48 hours, and it measured the acidity in two ways: How often stomach acid flowed back into the lower esophagus and the Degree of acidity during the test period. However, the test was of no consequence for me, because the capsule detached from my esophagus and no information was retrieved.

The diagnosis: Barrett's esophagus, again, with metaplasia but no dysplasia. This time was different. I was acutely aware of the seriousness of the diagnosis and the treatment.

My doctor's recommendation was that I take two 40mg Pantoprazole tablets (big boys) daily. "Here we go again." I thought. After years of reading about acid reducers, I knew too, that PPI's were not without their consequences: they induce acid-related symptoms like heartburn, acid regurgitation and dyspepsia once treatment is withdrawn in healthy individuals and many others. Why did I even take this test if there was no new treatment? My gastroenterologist also recommended dietary changes, the same ones which were printed on a nice little pamphlet and that I had been following for years: eliminate spices, coffee, lie in an inclined position with your head elevated, don't lie flat of your back, eliminate fats, etc., and lose weight.

Too make things worse; I had a friend who suffered from GERD and had gone down this same path that I was currently traveling taking Prilosec for symptoms but no real treatment for the cause of GERD. Now, he is experiencing the side effects of the long-term use of the Prilosec. He can't get off the Prilosec. Getting off aggravates his condition. It appears the drugs led to "rebound acid hyper secretion," which is an increase in gastric acid secretion *above pre-treatment levels.* It is my understanding that his condition relates to an enzyme overproduction. And now, he is going to the Mayo clinic receiving treatments for side effects of the Prilosec. He shared his journey with me and out of an abundance of concern, pleaded with me not to get trapped into taking the acid reducers long term. My awareness was acute. His warning contributed to my heightening awareness just as my experience of all these years with GERD. So, I had a choice to make: continue taking the acid reducing PPI's (proton Pump Inhibitors) or not to continue taking them. There would be consequences for taking the pills or not taking the pills.

3 THE BREAKING POINT

This chapter tells of my realization of the inherent dangers to my health and life if I choose to continue Pantoprazole.

I stopped taking the PPI's . I also stopped eating for a little while, because digestion was too painful. Driven to the breaking point, I set out like a mad scientist, once again. Digging through every medical book and research review. Anything that I could get my hands on that I thought might provide me with some answers about the conflicting theories about the causes of acid reflux.   I profiled every person that I came in contact with who had suffered from reflux.   And, I found the answer in the most unexpected of places: In a blog about Medicine for the 21st Century, I stumbled upon a series of articles about heartburn by Chris Kresser. Chris is a doctor and author of "What Everybody Ought To Know (But Doesn't) About Heartburn & GERD". Dr. Kresser wrote: ". Acid reflux is caused by too little stomach acid not too much…" (Kresser, n.d.) Well, even though I had read this many times before, this time when I read it, a crazy little thought, ". What causes my gut to have too little acid?" went through my head. And, this thought took me down a path that led to Dr. Norm Robillard, Ph. D, Microbiologist and Nutritionist, almost immediately. He is the author of Heartburn Cured, A Carbohydrate Miracle. "…Intestinal gas is the root cause of acid reflux", he said. "Intestinal gas of concern is produced primarily from microbial metabolism of excess carbohydrates, because unlike fats and proteins, carbohydrates are more readily and more rapidly utilized by microbes resulting in significant volumes of intestinal gas. Both simple and complex carbohydrates can contribute to acid reflux and heartburn in susceptible individuals," says Dr. Robillard. This was my answer! It was inconsistent with the conventional wisdom and the medical doctrine, as well as the treatment and information that I received from my doctors over the years. It offered me hope. As a matter of fact, it was the opposite of what doctors had been telling me. But I was aware of the differing opinions in the profession for a long time but didn't know how to advocate.

But now, I don't have to take pills for relief. I have an "ace in the hole."

4 THE CURE

This chapter will tell you how to use the 4-Steps proposed by Dr. Robillard to eliminate acid reflux.

Cure acid reflux by reducing the consumption of excess dietary carbohydrates. That's it! Just cut carbs by 10 fold. According to Dr. Norm Robillard's Heartburn Cured: The Low Carb Miracle, these carbs are the root cause of GERD. He devised a Theory that turns conventional wisdom on its head: "Intestinal gas of concern is produced primarily from microbial metabolism of excess carbohydrates, because unlike fats and proteins, carbohydrates are more readily and more rapidly utilized by microbes resulting in significant volumes of intestinal gas. Both simple and complex carbohydrates can contribute to acid reflux and heartburn in susceptible individuals,"

After significant research, I found several other reports corroborating this new theory. * His theory was completely reasonable to me and I felt confident to try his suggested low carb approach. After all, I had followed the doctor's advice for over 20 years without success. Well, let's go on down to the next paragraph to get this new dramatic four-step approach that I used to maintain a normal healthy diet while reducing carbohydrate consumption enough to alleviate my symptoms of acid reflux.

5 THE FOUR-STEP APPROACH

In the first step, carbs, which are fuel for gas producing microbes, need to be significantly limited to ensure that heartburn is stopped. (Robillard, n.d.)

After stopping your reflux, steps two and three helps you gradually add back carbohydrates, using your symptoms, or lack of symptoms as your guide to determine your optimal level of carbohydrate intake that will allow you to remain symptom free

The last step permanent relief allows you to develop a maintenance diet that will enable you to control heartburn on a permanent basis.

Week 1- (25 gram Net daily intake of Carbs)

What will I eat? To begin this diet I needed to significantly reduce my carb intake. This first week is decompression because I had to greatly reducing the fuel that allows my intestinal microbes to produce gas. Robillard recommended limiting the total net carbs to 25 grams. This would ensure a drastic reduction in intestinal gas and resulting heartburn. According to Dr. Robillard, The western diet contains 250-350 carbs per day. Wow! This amounts to reducing my carb intake ten fold. I've lost over 20 pounds during the first four weeks.

As for my heartburn, I felt the difference in a few days. During this time I changed my metabolism and that of my *friends*, the gut microbes. As I changed my diet, according to Norm, I caused a shift in the biochemical pathways used by the microbes as they adapt to the decrease in carbohydrates and increase in proteins and fats. This caused shifts in the populations of different microbes in my intestines by changing the ratio of protein, fat, and carbohydrates. Some microbes will be equipped to live off my new diet. Some will not. A mini evolution has occurred in my gut and now I have a new but friendly population of microbes that will aid my digestive process and help supply my needed nutritional factors.

Week 2: Equilibrium (45 Grams of Carbohydrates Per Day)

After one week at 25 grams per day, my heartburn symptoms were totally absent and my digestive systems seems to be in equilibrium, that is from gas pressure. In week two I had very little gas. This means that most of the carbs that I consume are being fully absorbed and very little is being leftover for the microbes to use to produce intestinal gas (Dr. Robillard advises, If you still have symptoms, you may want to advance to 30-35 net carbs per day for an additional week). "Remember, your body does not need carbs as long as you are getting your calcium and taking a multiple vitamin supplement daily." (Robillard, n.d.)

If your heartburn has ceased, you can now continue raising your carbohydrate intake gradually by as much as 20 additional net carbs total per day as the plan prescribes.

The first thing that I had to do was to clean my pantry and my refrigerator. Goodbye, to coffee, diet colas, artificial sweeteners, dairy products, sweets, sugars, beans, rice, cereals, etc.

Week 3 (Testing the Waters: 75-100 grams net carbs per day)

"If after completing the second phase (45 grams net carbs per day), you are completely heartburn free, you can experiment with higher levels. Add more net carbs per day to find your upper limit (the highest level of net carbs per day that will leave you heartburn free). Keep in mind that you can never return to the days of excess carbs. Once you find your upper limit of net carbs per day, not only will your heartburn be a thing of the past, your overall health will improve dramatically, " according to Norm Robillard.

Week 4 (Permanent Relief- tailored net carb intake level that controls heartburn)

I kept my net carbohydrate levels below 40 grams per day. I have found that when I go just a little beyond 40g, I feel minor symptoms recur. 40-45g is my personal tolerance level to prevent heartburn and hold it at bay. Not to mention the significant weight loss that I have experienced. Remember, it is your symptoms and your tolerance levels that should guide your net carbohydrate level in your final maintenance level.

Gwendolyn L. White

6 BEGINNING A LOW CARBOHYDRATE DIET

In this section you will find menus to help you plan your first week. Be sure to implement a tracking tool to measure your daily carbohydrate intake. I cannot over emphasize how important a tracking tool is to your success. Do this for each meal! Each day! I used Calorie King to track my carbs and the following menus to reduce my daily consumption of carbohydrates. The Paleo Diet Cookbook was a resource in meal planning for my very low carb diet. The essential rules of the Paleo Diet are: all the lean meats, poultry, fish, seafood, fruits (except dried fruits, and vegetables (except potatoes and corn) you can consume. This may have been the first time in my life without eating grains and dairy products. I also forgo sugars, artificial sweeteners, diet drinks and processed foods. The breakfasts took a little while getting used to because they were the most different from what I was accustomed. But with GERD, I couldn't allow these differences to worry me. I've been used to a breakfast that was a high-carbohydrate meal including some sort of cereal (steel cut oats, milk, buttered toast, pancakes, etc.) with coffee every morning. But now my breakfast's meats are chicken breasts, fish and steak. My morning meals are typically high in protein and low in carbohydrate and fat and consist of slices of cold London broil or cold crab legs (leftover from last night's dinner), and half of a cantaloupe or a bowl of fresh strawberries. Each morning and night, I drank a cup of warm water with lemon juice. My heaviest meal was lunch and I eat my last meal around 3:00 P.M. Here is a sample of one week on a low carb diet looks like for me.

7 LOW CARBOHYDRATE MENUS

DAY 1 (Sample Menus for a low carb diet)

Breakfast: My Spicy Breakfast Burrito (sauté sweet onion & chopped garlic clove in olive oil until tender. Stir in red bell pepper, cumin, diced chicken and black pepper, cayenne pepper and mix well. Stir in beaten eggs with a spatula until cooked thoroughly, sprinkle with black pepper. Wrap tightly in lettuce leaves.) and Youth berry Tea brewed w/filtered water.

Lunch: Oven Roasted Chicken Breast w/sautéed vegetables (onions, olive oil, Carrots)

Dinner: YellowPepper-Shrimppy Skewers (heat 2 tablespoons of extra virgin olive oil and add 3 pressed garlic cloves, add 1tsp paprika, 1 tsp. cayenne paper and tsp. dried dill; Sauté for a minute while stirring. Pour in ¼ cup white wine and simmer for two minutes. Add 20 medium shrimp, cover and simmer for 10 minutes. Drain excess liquid from shrimp. Spear shrimp, yellow bell pepper and tomato, alternating each until skewer is full. Drizzle each with fresh limejuice.

Snack: Egg Scoops (Remove the yolks from 4-Hard boiled Omega-3 Eggs and place in a mixing bowl. Add 1 tablespoon of coconut oil, 1-tablespoon of flaxseed oil, and 1 teaspoon of ground ginger. Smash together with a spoon and scoop back into each egg half. Sprinkle with paprika) Left Over Chicken Breast w/sautéed vegetables (onions, olive oil, Carrots)

DAY 2

Breakfast: 2 eggs w/(spinach, chopped basil, freshly ground black pepper sautéed in olive oil) folded into eggs, garnished with thin avocado slices, and Orange Blossom Tea brewed w/filtered water.

Lunch: Salmon Filet, w/salad field greens, walnuts, sliced cherry tomatoes, purple onion, baby carrots, lemon juice and olive oil.

Dinner: Turkey w/Asparagus Spears (Wrap one slice of roast turkey breast around each steamed asparagus spear. Heat one tablespoon of olive oil in a cast iron skillet; place the spears in the skillet. Cover and cook until turkey is nicely brown on each side.) Serve with Butternut Squash.

Snack: Cherry tomatoes

DAY 3

Breakfast: 2 eggs Scrambled and a cup of Youth berry Tea brewed w/filtered water.

Lunch: Oven Roasted Chicken Breast w/sautéed vegetables (onions, olive oil, Carrots).

Dinner: Spinach Salad w/ Strawberries (Combine 4-cups torn spinach leaves with 1cup hulled and quartered strawberries in a salad bowl. In a small jar combine 2 Tablespoons. Extra Virgin Olive oil and lime juice and shake well. Toss with spinach and berries and sprinkle with cashews.)

Snack: Egg Scoops (Remove the yolks from 4-Hard boiled Omega-3 Eggs and place in a mixing bowl. Add 1 tablespoon of coconut oil, 1-tablespoon of flaxseed oil, and 1 teaspoon of ground ginger. Smash together with a spoon and scoop back into each egg half. Sprinkle with paprika) Left Over Chicken Breast w/sautéed vegetables (onions, olive oil, Carrots)

Day 4

Breakfast: Scrambled egg and a warm cup of Orange Blossom Tea.

Lunch: Salad (Romaine Lettuce, Grape Tomatoes, bell pepper, Purple Onion, Boiled eggs, Lemon Juice, Olive Oil and Chicken Breast)

Dinner: Chicken Breast Filet, Sautéed (onions, tomato, Basil, mushrooms) Turnip Greens and Baked Sweet Potato.

Snack: Egg Scoops (Remove the yolks from 4-Hard boiled Omega-3 Eggs and place in a mixing bowl. Add 1 tablespoon of coconut oil, 1-tablespoon of flaxseed oil, and 1 teaspoon of ground ginger. Smash together with a spoon and scoop back into each egg half. Sprinkle with paprika) Left Over Chicken Breast w/sautéed vegetables (onions, olive oil, Carrots)

DAY 5

Breakfast: Cooked Shrimp & egg dish (sauté minced yellow onion in olive oil and combine with beat eggs. Add cooked shrimp, dill, and basil and mix thoroughly until eggs are wet but not completely cooked. Stir in artichoke hearts and finish cooking.) Served with Warm Tea

Lunch: Bok Choy and Braised Leeks with garlic (Loren Cordain, n.d.). Baked Sweet Potato and Blackened Salmon filet: Salad (Spinach, purple onion, celery, bell pepper, cherry tomatoes, olive oil and lemon juice).

Dinner: Salad (Romaine Lettuce, spinach, Grape Tomatoes, bell pepper, Purple Onion, Boiled eggs, Lemon Juice, Olive Oil and oven roasted Chicken Breast)

Snack: Egg Scoops (Remove the yolks from 4-Hard boiled Omega-3 Eggs and place in a mixing bowl. Add 1 tablespoon of coconut oil, 1-tablespoon of flaxseed oil, and 1 teaspoon of ground ginger. Smash together with a spoon and scoop back into each egg half. Sprinkle with paprika) Left Over Chicken Breast w/sautéed vegetables (onions, olive oil, Carrots)

Day 6

Breakfast: Scrambled Egg and tea,

Lunch: Salad (Romaine Lettuce, Grape Tomatoes, bell pepper, Purple Onion, Boiled eggs, Lemon Juice, Olive Oil).

Dinner: Smokey Southern Style Collards (4-ounces diced roasted turkey breast/sautéed & charred diced yellow onion & garlic w/thyme and basil) mixed with coarsely chopped collard greens w/ stems removed, stirred and cook together)

Snack: Egg Scoops (Remove the yolks from 4-Hard boiled Omega-3 Eggs and place in a mixing bowl. Add 1 tablespoon of coconut oil, 1-tablespoon of flaxseed oil, and 1 teaspoon of ground ginger. Smash together with a spoon and scoop back into each egg half. Sprinkle with paprika) Left Over Chicken Breast w/sautéed vegetables (onions, olive oil, Carrots)

DAY 7

Breakfast: My Breakfast Burrito (sauté sweet onion & chopped garlic clove in olive oil until tender. Stir in red bell pepper, cumin, diced chicken and black pepper and mix well then stir in beaten eggs with a spatula until cooked thoroughly, sprinkle with black pepper. Wrap tightly in lettuce leaves.)

Lunch: Braised Leeks with Garlic (Paleo, n.d) (Loren Cordain, n.d.). Oven fried chicken breast and spaghetti squash.

Dinner: Salad (Romaine Lettuce, spinach, Grape Tomatoes, bell pepper, Purple Onion, Boiled eggs, Lemon Juice, Olive Oil and oven roasted Chicken Breast)

8 PLAN FOR SUCCESS

A Few Tips

I take a multi vitamin and calcium supplement daily and drink lots of water. I eat fresh veggies at every meal, including breakfast, folding chopped scallions, avocado slices and diced tomatoes into my omelets, which are made with omega 3 enriched eggs. I eat one sweet potato on most days (I just like them) and stay away from peas and green beans, which are legumes. Otherwise, I enjoy the incredibly healthy foods: artichoke, asparagus, beet greens, beets, bell peppers, broccoli, Brussels sprouts, cabbage, carrots, cauliflower, celery, collards, cucumber, dandelion, eggplant, endive, green onions, kale, kohlrabi, lettuce, mushrooms, mustard greens, onions, parsley, parsnip, peppers, pumpkin, purslane, radish, rutabaga, seaweed, spinach, squash, sweet potatoes, Swiss chard, tomatillos, tomato, turnip greens, turnips, watercress, and yams.

Nuts and Seeds

I consume nuts modestly, especially walnuts. I learned that peanuts are legumes, not nuts, and were absolutely not on the Paleo Diet menu. Peanuts contain substances that rapidly enter our bloodstreams and can promote allergies, autoimmune diseases and hear disease (Loren Cordain, n.d.).

"Calorie King" and "Lose It" are great food tracker tools. They are easily downloaded to your iPhone or iPad. I have both tools on my iPhone and that makes them readily available for instant use anywhere and anytime. There exist many others similar applications out there. I use one or both of them daily to keep track of my daily net grams of carbohydrate intake or search for nutritional information; and check my progress with weight gain or loss. Each of these tools has an amazing search component that I use to determine the carbohydrate content of any particular food item. I log in daily to record my meals, exercises, etc. These apps are on my iPhone and therefore, handy for immediate use. I used both because I started out with "lose it" and some foods were not in its data bank. Calorie King provided more search results and nutritional value information but not the sophisticated meal planning of Lose It. But now there is a newer version on Calorie King and it is just as amazing. So now I am using Calorie King. The only application that I use more is my dictionary. The information on calorie king was more extensive.

9 FINALLY, FREE FROM ACID REFLUX

For the first time in my adult life, I am free of acid reflux and acid reducing medications. I realize that I cannot ever go back to my old habits of 300 grams of carbs per day. Altering the habits of a lifetime is not easy. I am finally free of acid reflux and it's symptoms which have plagued me for years. I am writing this book for acid reflux and GERD suffers to share the consequences of allowing acid reflux to go untreated for a period of time. The miracle of the low carb diet is the most important take away from my story. It allows you to stop the use omeprazole (Prilosec), pantoprazole (Protonix), syntax (ranitidine), and all other proton pomp inhibitors (PPI), if you haven't gotten addicted to them. A few lifestyle changes have enabled me to live life free of acid reflux pills. The low carb approach is my ace in the hole. Knowing that I can control the conditions that have been devastating to my health; and to do it without using drugs is gratifying. Losing the unwanted excess weight was an added bonus. I believe that this approach has also alleviated other health issues that may have been associated with acid reflux. My breathing feels better! My joints that were once afflicted with arthritic pain don't ache anymore, energy is high and I feel good. I am finally free.

10 REFERENCES

Kresser, C. (Medicine for the 21st C. (n.d.). What Everybody Ought To Know (But Doesn't) About Heartburn & GERD. *My name is Chris Kresser, and I'm a licensed acupuncturist and practitioner of integrative medicine.* Retrieved March 1, 2013, from http://chriskresser.com/what-everybody-ought-to-know-but-doesnt-about-heartburn-gerd

Loren Cordain, P. D. and N. S. (n.d.). *The Paleo Diet Cookbook* (2011th ed.). Hoboken, New Jersey: John Wiley & Sons, Inc. Hoboken, New Jersey. Retrieved from http://thepaleodiet.com/healthy-eating/dr-cordains-interview-with-lx-magazine/

Ness-Jensen, E., Lindam, A., Lagergren, J., & Hveem, K. (2012). Changes in prevalence, incidence and spontaneous loss of gastro-esophageal reflux symptoms: a prospective population-based cohort study, the HUNT study. *Gut, 61*(10), 1390–7. Retrieved from http://gut.bmj.com/content/early/2011/12/15/gutjnl-2011-300715.abstract

Robillard, N. P. (n.d.). *Heartburn Cured - The Low Carb Miracle.*

Why Stomach Acid Is Good For You DR. WRIGHT'S PRODUCTS. (n.d.). Retrieved April 13, 2013, from http://www.tahomadispensary.com/store/4275!347/Why+Stomach+Acid+Is+Good+For+You

Why You Should Get Off Prescription Acid-Reducing Drugs ASAP! (n.d.). Retrieved April 26, 2013, from http://articles.mercola.com/sites/articles/archive/2009/09/05/why-you-should-get-off-prescription-acid-reducing-drugs-asap.aspx

Dr. Michal and Mary Dan Eades (2009). The most predictable beneficial results.

Adkins, Robert (n.d). Adkins for Life by Dr. Robert Adkins, Retrieved April 13, 3013

Tom Cowan – San Francisco based doctor (n.d)

Paleo Diet Cookbook(Loren Cordain, n.d.)

(Wright, J. (n.d.) "Why Stomach Acid Is Good For You.)

("Why You Should Get Off Prescription Acid-Reducing Drugs ASAP!," n.d.)

My name is Gwendolyn L. White. I was born in Pine Bluff, Arkansas and lived there for forty years. I received a BS Degree in mathematics from the University of Arkansas at Pine Bluff, formerly AM&N College. I received a M.Ed. in Mathematics Education from Georgia State University. I am retired mathematics teacher..

My teaching career began at Watson Chapel High School in Pine Bluff, Arkansas, where I taught HS Mathematics for 19 years. During this time I participated in STRIVE, a summer lab program that paired teachers with scientists. This program allowed teachers to work side by side with National Center for Toxicological Research (NCTR) scientists to gain research experience. During this summer program, with the assistance of national scientists, I worked to develop a computer software programs that was used in local school classrooms.

In 1992, I moved to Atlanta, Georgia and began teaching H.S. Mathematics in DeKalb County. For the next eight years, I enjoyed being a Gift Alumnus with a cohort of Georgia teachers. I participated in several summer initiatives sponsored by Georgia State University at: Georgia Tech, Phillips Exeter Academy and MCI.

In 2002, I relocated to Fairfax County, VA where I worked in the Fairfax county public schools teaching for 7 years. After this time, I returned to Atlanta, Ga. and I taught eight years at Druid Hills High School and retired in December 2012.

I was married for 19 years and have two daughters, two son-in-laws and five grand children. I enjoy reading, writing, planning, and traveling (got to do this). I have written a few non-fiction short stories as well as some poetry. I am currently delving into the World Wide Web, studying web designing and the digital world of marketing.